Start Here!

How to have Success with *ANY* Diet and Fitness Program

By Tony Simoneli

Eloquent Books
New York, New York

Eloquent Books
An imprint of AEG Publishing Group
845 Third Avenue, 6th Floor - 6016
New York, NY 10022
www.eloquentbooks.com

ISBN 978-1-60860-421-0

Printed in the United States of America

Book Design: Linda W. Rigsbee

Dedication

This book is dedicated to my father Jim who has inspired me to live healthy and be free. To my brother Raymond from whom I've learned what it means to be brave and persevere.

Table of Contents

Content Disclaimer

This content is for informational purposes only. The Content is not intended to be a substitute for professional medical advice, diagnosis, or treatment. Always seek the advice of your physician or other qualified health provider with any questions you may have regarding a medical condition.

Never disregard professional medical advice or delay in seeking it because of something you have read in this book – Start Here! How to have Success with Any Diet or Fitness Program. Reliance on any information provided by the book or any Company Affiliate with the book is solely at your own risk.

About the Author

At 39 years young I've been involved with many types of sports and exercise during my life, following in the footsteps of my dad. Growing up with a young dad who was interested in his health, I was given the opportunity to try a large variety of sports like racing bikes, power lifting, American kenpo karate, football, soccer and playing rugby until I joined the Air Force and went to Desert Storm.

Along with sports, my dad seeded my interest in exercise by teaching me what he knew and bringing me to health clubs as a kid. I became fascinated with how the body works and marveled at what an incredible machine the human body is. To this day when I watch a TV show about engineers trying to produce robots and machines to replicate simple human movements I'm left with a sense of admiration in how nature has overcome these obstacles. I can't help but reflect on how ingenious nature is. I'm also constantly a student. After all, we, the human race, are constantly learning more about ourselves as we press forward in life. I'm always interested in learning more and because of this I've adapted my knowledge, not only with my clients over the years but with myself as well. Now considered middle-aged, I've personally gone through the aches and pains of getting older as well as controlling my weight. I gained fifty pounds in a relatively short time after getting married. As a person who 'practices what he preaches', this was a challenge for me to prove it. I've now returned to what I weighed in my twenties, although maybe not quite as muscular as I was then, but I feel great and I'm now living proof to the methods that I've been teaching others for over ten years.

My Experience

I have been nationally certified as a Personal Trainer from the National Academy of Sports Medicine (NASM) since 1998, including additional certifications in Optimal Performance Training with NASM as well as Nutrition from Apex Fitness. Although I'm able to instruct in a vast array of training methods, my specialties are balance and stability training, which includes focus on the smaller muscle groups that support the joints. In addition, I work on posture correction that focuses on correcting muscle imbalances, which pull the body out of correct alignment and change its center of gravity. This imbalance can cause many physical ailments, including chronic joint pain as well as the very prevalent chronic low back pain. In the years since obtaining my certification, I have taken many related classes and workshops as well as reading countless books and publications to continue my education.

My work experience includes various management roles in health clubs, including Fitness Director. I've also been a sales person for fitness equipment, have taught multiple workshops and classes on fitness and designed and operated a children's fitness program that I called C.O.R.E. 4Kids.

My Personal Philosophy

To continue my education and grow, physically, emotionally and spiritually while bettering the lives of others.

How you can benefit from this book

In part the health club industry depends upon the yearly cycle of new members that allow them to stay in business. You know the story. In January mass amounts of well-meaning people flock to the health clubs to begin a New Year's resolution of fitness and fat loss, only to find by March or April about eighty percent drop out, but *continue to pay for the membership for the next year or two.* The clubs need to maintain a steady stream of revenue; this is why most health clubs today lock you into a one or two year contract. One day I was discussing this phenomenon with my colleagues. We analyzed why people quit their resolutions instead of completing their goals and narrowed it down to what we felt were the two main reasons:

✦ **First Scenario** – Many who have joined a health club are new and likely clueless to fitness and the health club itself. You flock to the clubs and begin exercise programs of varying sorts with every intention of fulfilling your dream of a healthy lifestyle. However, you may be timid and apprehensive because you're not sure where to start. You are most likely self-conscious about how you look and about your lack of experience. You soon get overwhelmed with the mass amounts of information that you've picked up in regards to correct techniques or the quickest pathways to success. Most of this information is false or a fad, given freely by well-meaning "*experts*" or it's something you saw on TV. You soon get frustrated, more self-conscious, sore, tired, and eventually give up, thinking 'this is too difficult'. Am I getting warm?

✦ **Second Scenario** – You are a person who used to be active and healthy, but have "let your self go" over the years and now you're trying to return to your old routines. You've convinced yourself that you still "got it" (and you might not be far off) and you try to keep up with the seasoned club members or athletes only to over-do-it, getting very sore, tired, and never show up again. Perhaps you're even embarrassed at making the attempt in the first place. Am I on the right track?

I find most everyone will agree that quality personal training would be very beneficial and it is the best way to achieve your goals, but it can get expensive, costing hundreds, even thousands of dollars for a trainer that *really* knows what they are doing. Good news though: this book will fill in the gaps by providing you with the quality education and training that you're looking for at an *extremely* affordable price. Why do I bother you may ask? It's because I'm a teacher and dedicated to educating others on how to develop a healthy lifestyle - not profits, fads, or gimmicks. I love what I do! I have filtered through all the fads and hype that you find with fitness so you can learn the *true* fundamentals that will help you to succeed with *any* diet or fitness program that you wish to begin (or should I say complete?). Over the years I've found that some of my clients didn't even know what a repetition or a set was and this is really basic information. If you don't know either, don't worry; I'll explain it to you soon. I've also made this book very easy to understand so you can begin *enjoying* the healthy lifestyle that you've envisioned for yourself right away. With this book I've purposely stuck to the basics for two reasons:

1) There are a lot of people out there that don't know the basics and I want to enable you to make the correct foundation steps in order for you to quickly absorb and put to practice what you are reading.

2) As you get more adapted to creating your healthy lifestyle, you will get more excited and begin to gather additional information, on your own and at the speed that is right for you. It's my belief that in this way, you will retain *more* information - faster. We all do when it's something we enjoy!

A Little History of Fitness

Back in the 1950s and 1960s health clubs were called gyms and they catered mainly to men who were training for specific goals such as bodybuilding (which was in its infant stages), power lifting, or to enhance sports performance.

When the 1970s came around, going to the gym became an active outlet and a hip social environment for most everyone, no matter their fitness level or ability. Some didn't even exercise; they were there just to be a part of the "happening scene". A lot of gyms during this time even had a bar serving beer and wine! It was also a time when exercise was realized to be a way to alter your physical appearance - just in time for a generation that became conscious about how they looked. However, because "working out" was still a new concept, many people needed guidance.

The "expert" was usually the guy who was the strongest or who looked the biggest or the most fit. These people became the unofficial personal trainers at a time when there wasn't such a thing as personal trainers, only athletic coaches. Because these "trainers" basically had no education in regards to either training or the human body, they mostly put others through the same routines they performed themselves. With steroids becoming more popular, some of these routines were very difficult for those not using them, especially if the person giving the guidance was.

During the 1980s our lives became more and more automated along with an increased demand for our attendance at work. We had less and less time for physical leisure activities like we did in the past. So it's not surprising that as far back as 1985 the *International Obesity Task Force* announced obesity to be an oncoming epidemic.

The 1990's ushered in a profound change in fitness. This decade brought us a more dynamic look at how the body functions, which led to further advancements with fitness equipment. These changes allowed equipment to move more like the body naturally does in everyday life, which ultimately made the equipment more comfortable to use. *Precore* is a great example with the invention of the elliptical trainer in 1995.

During this decade, personal training was now being recognized as a serious profession and an excellent revenue source for health clubs. With our increased awareness of a healthy lifestyle and its associated benefits we started to demand more knowledgeable training professionals. Companies, along with those who took their personal training job seriously, strived for better regulation on becoming a personal trainer. Today companies are currently working to get personal trainer's licensed by the state like contractors.

Obesity in America...

Regardless of the proven benefits of physical activity, more than sixty percent of American adults do not get enough physical activity to provide health benefits. More than twenty-five percent are not active *at all* in their leisure time.

...Still on the rise

Here is a statement published by the *National Center for Health Statistics*:

Obesity continued to increase dramatically during the late 1990s for Americans of all ages, with nearly one-third of all adults now classified as obese, according to new data from the 1999-2000 National Health and Nutrition Examination Survey published today in the Journal of the American Medical Association.

Data from the most recent NHANES survey shows that the percentage of adults aged twenty years and over who are overweight or obese has increased to 66.3 percent.

Wow! All of this regardless of the increased awareness of health and exercise and the benefits it provides.

The Problem May Be Worse For Children

A few years back I developed and operated a children's fitness program I named Creative Obesity Recreation Exercises for kids or **C.O.R.E. 4Kids**. While doing research to gain more knowledge in developing the program I came across some scary statistics in regards to the health of children these days:

+ The latest available stats for children that are obese are from 2003-2004 and are as follows: age 2-5: 13.9 percent, age 6-11: 18.8 percent and age 12-19: 17.4 percent. This means that 16.3 percent of children ages 2 to 19 are considered *obese*, which is at or above the 95th percentile of the 2000 BMI-for-age growth charts, whereas from 1971 to 1974 the numbers were only 4 percent.

+ From 1979 to 2000, health care costs for obesity related conditions in 6-7 year olds *alone* increased from $35 million to $127 million.

+ Every week children watch an average of forty-two hours of television and play seven hours of video games. That's a workweek with overtime!

+ Fewer than twenty percent of children get twenty minutes of vigorous activity every day. In fact, fewer than twenty-five percent report getting half an hour of *any type* of physical activity every day.

+ In 1991, forty-two percent of the nation's school children participated in physical education programs. By 1999, that number had dropped to twenty-one percent!

I've learned from the *National Center for Health Statistics* that the U.S. economy is currently spending over $100,000,000,000 *every year* for conditions caused by being overweight and obese. Yes folks, that's *one hundred billion*! Being overweight means you have a Body Mass Index (BMI) of 25 to 29.9 percent. Obese means you have a BMI of 30 to 34.9 percent.

You have the power to combat this with exercise and you don't even have to exercise much. A *little* regular physical activity substantially reduces the risk of health related problems like coronary heart disease (the nation's leading cause of death), stroke, colon cancer, diabetes, and high blood pressure - just to name a few. Regular exercise also helps to control weight; contributes to healthy bones, muscles and joints; reduces falls among older adults; helps to relieve the pain of arthritis; reduces symptoms of anxiety and depression, and is associated with fewer hospitalizations, physician visits, and medications. But you already knew this, right?

Even though there are approximately 26,830 health and fitness clubs in the U.S. (according to the International Health, Racquet & Sportsclub Association – IHRSA - 2005) they still only enroll about twelve percent of the possible market. Physical activity doesn't need be strenuous to be beneficial. People of all ages benefit from participating in regular moderate-intensity physical activity such as twenty minutes of *brisk* walking three or more times a week. Simple.

One thing to remember is that exercise should be fun and enjoyable! It's a pet peeve of mine to hear clients or friends whine, "Uhhh I have to go work out". It shouldn't be something you **HAVE** to do – it should be something you **WANT** to do.

This is part of my philosophy with this book; enjoy the time you spend while exercising. Make it the time you get to sift through your day, or the break you may need from the hustle and bustle of the family and everyday life. Then, when you do go exercise, you can tell everyone; "I *get* to go exercise now!"

Better Than a Personal Trainer?

There is a lot to be said for working in-person with a quality fitness trainer. However, the majority of people who work with a trainer miss out on a very important element. While exercising with their trainer, clients are being corrected or asked to make adjustments here, turn a little more there, or tighten up a bit more and so on. Clients will listen to what the trainer is telling them and then continue through the motions, which are usually coupled with a conversation about their day or events.

What happens after they've completed their sessions and they are on their own is that they can't remember most of what the trainer was teaching them! Clients subconsciously made the changes that the trainer would give and went on chatting, or thinking about work or kids and so forth. They now scratch their heads wondering what to do. They seem to have forgotten how to do the exercises they have been doing for weeks!

I estimate about seventy percent of clients forget sixty to eighty-five percent of everything they were taught. They were too busy concentrating on other things and didn't focus on what they were paying a trainer for in the first place - training. However, in their defense, trainers do provide an enormous amount of information and it can take awhile to absorb everything. Good trainers spend years learning what they know.

Now, some clients don't mind not remembering. They just want someone there to push them through a routine or listen to them talk about life (trainers can sometimes become psychologists for some clients). However, they are usually the people that have the means to pay for a trainer over and over again. Once clients realize they don't remember how to carry out the exercises on their own, they begin asking the trainer a ton of questions every time they get the chance. Trainers who are running a successful business try to accommodate as much as possible but they are trying to *run a business* and they only get paid if they can sign up more sessions. If the trainer has some free time they will be more than happy to answer questions. At most of the larger health clubs they usually have trainers scheduled during the day specifically to go around the club and answer questions or lend a hand if a member needs it. This is called Floor Time.

By using a *quality* training book like this one, you'll tend to retain the knowledge better. You will also make the most out of your money because don't have to pay for a trainer but have important information at your fingertips. You will have to really think about what you are doing and concentrate on where your hand goes, or when to breathe, or how to position your feet. Likewise, you can always refer back to a chapter as needed. It's during this time you develop your questions, as you are doing the exercise, instead of after the fact. The level of improvement seen in clients is tremendous! Are you getting excited yet?

Great! Let's Get Started!

Dieting

There are a myriad of diet plans out there and this topic could warrant a whole book by itself. I'm not going to go into a lot of descriptions on the various diets because the fact of the matter is, a large percentage of these diets are fad-based and not really healthy for you. Most of them will only work for a short while because they put such a shock to the body. Most people gain the weight back. Some gain even more!

Instead, I will relate to you the fundamentals of proper nutrition. This way, if you go exploring diet plans, you will be better armed in knowing what these plans are talking about and have a foundation on which to base your decision.

Introduction to Nutrition

One thing to keep in mind is that the human body is a very remarkable machine that has been around for a long time. Your body *knows* what it's doing. What throws most of us off is the human quest to make life easier. Because of automation we have more leisure time available and, because of automation, we spend the bulk of this time being physically *inactive*. Thus we tend to become lazy and, for some, when we reach that critical point, we look for the lazy solution.

No fad diet will make you healthy by itself and as I've said before I'm doubtful it would give you real long-term results. You *have* to include an exercise program to have lasting success and your exercise program doesn't even have to be that strenuous. Our bodies are designed to have exercise. Remember, we've spent hundreds of thousands of years as hunters and gatherers. We have only lost our way in approximately the last hundred years when the Industrial Revolution really started to take off. We no longer have to work for our food as we did in the past. Nowadays it only takes a short drive to the store or fast food joint. Our bodies are going to adapt to this change but Mother Nature runs on a different timeline than what has become the norm for us. I'll explain how to make the changes safely in a bit.

Most diet programs out there will claim theirs is the best way to achieve your goals and they will throw all kinds of scientific terms at you and maybe even have a Doctor endorse their product to sound more impressive. Do you want to know why they make all this effort?

They're trying to make money!

The way to lose body fat is simple – very simple if you do what's necessary. It's called the **Law of Thermal Dynamics** – You lose weight if you burn more calories than you consume. That's it.

You can watch all the infomercials you want, explaining in very technical terms the details of how and why the body will do certain things with their pill, drink or style of eating that they recommend but most won't work. Think back to all the different diets that you've seen come and go over the years or that you may have tried already. If they were that good in the first place, what happened to them? It's my beliefs that if they were great to begin with, they would be taught in schools, not disappear.

Have you ever heard of the **K.I.S.S** principle?

Keep

It

Simple

Silly

Don't try to make things more difficult than they are. The body works best this way. Don't get confused with the hype from people trying to make money. When counting your calories here are some basics that can go a long way:

One gram of protein = four calories,

One gram of carbohydrate = four calories

One gram of fat = nine calories

One ounce of alcohol = seven calories.

You want to watch your calories but you'll also want to watch what kind of calories you are putting into your body. I'll discuss this more in a bit.

Note: Alcohol is an "empty calorie". Meaning, it has no nutritional value at all but it will contribute to the ebb and flow of your body composition. If the alcoholic beverage also contains carbohydrates (sugars) then the calories for this beverage will be even higher. For example, according to Forbes.com in the health section a margarita can contain as much as seven hundred plus calories per drink! Drink only three of these and you almost used up your whole day's worth of calories! This, of course, depends on the way it's made and the size of the drink.

Protein

Protein, along with carbohydrates and fats, are part of a group called Macronutrients. These are the basic components of your nutrition. Protein is what your body uses to build and repair tissues and cell structures. It also synthesizes hormones and enzymes. Your body can use protein for energy, but will *only do so when your body has insufficient carbohydrates* in its diet. Think about that last line when considering a popular diet that is making the rounds.

Protein is made from *amino acids* linked together. Amino acids are classified into two categories:

Essential Amino Acids

Essential amino acids are small bits of protein that cannot be manufactured in the body (or they are manufactured in insufficient amounts). They must be obtained through food or supplementation. Protein can come from any variety of sources such as animal products, fermented soy, any variety of beans and some grains.

Non-Essential Amino Acids

These are amino's that are manufactured within the body. They do not require you to consume them.

In order for your body to digest and utilize protein, it must be broken down into amino acids.

Satiety is the feeling of being full. Protein has been shown to increase satiety and thus decrease the desire for food intake (this is a big factor in popular protein diets).

Negative Side Effects Associated with a Chronic High-Protein Diet

A high-protein diet is one where protein constitutes more than thirty percent of your total caloric intake. This can lead to some negative side effects like:

+ Calcium depletion (osteoporosis)
+ Fluid imbalance
+ Slower metabolism (the opposite of your weight-loss goals)
+ Weight rebound
+ Loss of energy

Protein Intake Recommendations

Endurance Athlete – 1.4 grams per 3.09 pounds of bodyweight per day.

Bodybuilder – 1.0 gram per 2.20 pounds bodyweight per day.

Recreational Athlete – 1.0 gram per 2.20 pounds bodyweight per day.

Note: If you are pregnant, you will have a need for extra protein in your diet. Consult with your Doctor for the recommended guidelines based on your particular needs.

Carbohydrates

Carbohydrates (also called carbs) are compounds commonly classified as:

+ Sugars (simple carbohydrates)

+ Starches (complex carbohydrates)

+ Fiber

All carbohydrates are made up of sugars. Although there are a number of different types of sugars, in the body all carbohydrates are converted from sugar to glucose, the body's *preferred* energy source.

Glucose is the main sugar present in many foods. Some foods contain different types of sugars, such as fructose in fruit, and lactose in milk. Most sugars are digested, absorbed and converted to glucose. Some cannot be digested and we call this fiber.

Simple Carbohydrates

Simple carbohydrates are smaller molecules of sugar. Individual sugar molecules themselves – glucose, fructose and galactose –

are called monosaccharides. When you have two sugar molecules bonded together they are called disaccharides. They are digested quickly because the individual sugars are ready to be absorbed immediately. Plus the digestive enzymes that break food down for you have easy access to the bonds that hold the molecules together. With simple sugars you could say that most of the work has already been done for you!

However, their rapid absorption *increases* the chances of sugar being converted to fat, especially if there are large quantities consumed at one time. Processed foods like cake, pastries, biscuits, chocolate and table sugar, to name only a few, are easily converted to fat because they contain much more sugar than the body needs. This is why you should avoid processed foods altogether. I know they are quicker to prepare or grab off the shelf but they will lead to a quicker failure with your health goals.

Because our cells usually do not require such a large amount of energy at one time, the sugar must either be converted to glycogen (sugar storage within cells) or converted to fat. However cells can only store a limited amount of glycogen. Foods loaded with simple carbohydrates will contribute greatly to fat stores unless you have enough physical activity to burn it off. Remember the Law of Thermal Dynamics?

Natural foods, like fruit, contain naturally occurring simple sugars (fructose) but, because the amount of sugar is low, there's less chance for it to be converted to fat. Plus many fruits are high in fiber, which helps slow digestion, thus limiting the flood of sugar into the body when it's not needed.

Complex Carbohydrates

Complex carbohydrates, or starches, are sugars bonded together to form a chain. Digestive enzymes have to work much harder to access the bonds and break the chain into individual sugars for absorption through the intestines. For this reason, digestion of complex carbohydrates takes longer. The slow absorption of these sugars provides us with a steady stream of energy and limits the amount of sugar converted into fat. Examples of these types of sugars are potatoes, rice, bread and pasta.

Fiber

Fiber is an elongated, thread-like structure in fruits, vegetables and grains that cannot be digested. They help grab the gunk in your intestines and keep them working properly. The benefits of fiber include:

+ Lowers incidences of heart disease and certain types of cancer, including colon cancer

+ Provides bulk to the diet

+ Increases satiety (the feeling of being full)

+ Prevents constipation and establishes bowel regularity

+ Aides in the prevention of bacterial infections

- ✦ Helps retain the health of the digestive-tract muscles

- ✦ Regulates the body's absorption of glucose (sugar)

Note: High-fiber meals have been shown to exert regulatory effects on blood-glucose (sugar) levels for up to five hours after eating.

Pre-Exercise Intake

Remember, carbs are your body's preferred source of energy. It's recommended to eat a high-carb meal two to three hours before activities that will last one hour or longer. This will allow you to fully digest and empty your stomach. If this isn't possible for you due to time constraints, then a liquid meal-replacement formula may be used, or better yet a smaller meal eaten closer to the time of your workout, such as oatmeal. Just remember to watch your serving size.

Carbs and Body Composition

Carbohydrates should make up the *highest* percentage of your macronutrient calories when you are attempting either to lose fat or gain muscle.

I know some of you are feeling defensive right now if you're on a high-protein diet plan, but as I've said earlier, the body is just not set up to run on such high doses of protein.

For most moderately active adults, your diet should consist of about fifty to sixty percent carbohydrates. The satiating value with carbs, especially complex carbs, when trying to lose weight is very helpful. Protein should *only* make up about twenty-five to thirty percent of your diet. The last ten to fifteen percent is left for fats.

Fats

Fats are often the "bad word" when it comes to dieting. However, fats are needed as part of your healthy diet as there are many benefits associated with them. You just have to know the good, the bad and the ugly. The fats that we want to discuss are lipids, which are further classified as triglycerides.

The Bad (also ugly)

Saturated fat – This is the fat that becomes hard and whitish in color at room temperature and is found mostly in animal products. Think about a cooked steak you've left out for a while. It's that yucky white stuff you scrape off when you go to reheat it later. Saturated fat is the stuff that is implicated in the increase of LDL or "bad" cholesterol.

When shopping look for the leanest cuts that you can find. Most meat departments will even trim the meat for you at no cost if you ask them. Grilling meat is the preferred way to cook it. The fat will drip off into the bottom of the grill allowing the steak to become healthier to eat.

The Good

Unsaturated fat – is implicated in HDL or "good" cholesterol. This can be found in products like olive oil, canola oil and almond oil. Mono-unsaturated fat is a double bond in its chain. Poly-unsaturated fat has more than one in its double-bonded chain. These are found in peanuts, macadamia nuts, safflower oil and corn oil. Don't worry if this is starting to sound overwhelming just remember that unsaturated fat is good.

The benefits of these fats are:

+ Provides energy

+ Transports fat-soluble vitamins like A, D, E and K

+ Provides regulation and excretion of nutrients in the cells

+ Provides organ protection

+ Initiates the release of the hormone cholecystokinin, which is a hormone that signals satiety (feeling full)

A recap of what your suggested macronutrient intake should be are as follows:

+ Carbohydrates should make up the bulk of your food intake at 50-60 percent

+ Protein should only be about 25-30 percent of your diet

+ 10 to 15 percent is left for fats

And don't forget the Law of Thermal Dynamics – You lose body fat when you burn more calories than you take in.

Changing Your Body Composition

Measure your Body Composition – Not your Weight

Your total weight is a combination of bone, ligaments, tendons, organs, fluids, muscle and of course fat. When you gain or lose weight due to either a fitness program or neglecting your health, then your overall weight will change, as well as the ratio of these elements to one another. The term body composition is defined as the relationship between all the lean tissue within the body and the fat.

One of the most difficult, yet important, concepts that will help you with your journey to a healthy lifestyle is **it's not what you weigh, but the relationship of your lean mass to your fat mass**.

It's not uncommon for a person to begin a fitness program and not see a decrease in weight while experiencing a decrease in inches at the waist – which is most likely your goal. Sometimes you might even *gain* a pound or two. The point I want to make is that you shouldn't be so concerned with your weight as long as you are losing the inches. Men don't usually have a problem with constantly checking the scale but women tend to focus only on their weight because society and the media have made such a mental impact.

Muscle weighs three times more than fat per volume, and as you gain lean muscle (not necessarily bulk) as you exercise, you can be smaller physically but weigh more. The distinction between being "over-weight" and "over-fat" is important to learn here. As an active person, when you exercise regularly, you will gain more muscle from your activities, and thus possibly gain weight, but you'll lose inches and body fat which allows you to fit into your "skinny jeans" and that's the real goal right?

Likewise, if you maintain your current daily calorie intake but don't add any more physical activity, the result is probably the body composition you have now. I want to give you a link to *The Department of Health and Human Services* BMI (Body Mass Index) calculator to see where you are currently. Keep in mind however that you should visit your doctor or a personal trainer to get the most accurate reading: (http://www.cdc.gov/nccdphp/dnpa/bmi/calc-bmi.htm). This will give you a better idea as to what you really should lose.

Now that you have an understanding of your body composition, I want to explain some of the ways you can change it. The old motto of three square meals a day isn't the best way to eat. It's recommended that you eat smaller meals more frequently – about four to six times per day. It may sound like a lot, but I'm willing to bet that if you tracked your current eating habits, including junk food snacks, you will probably find that you are already are doing this.

An example would be; 7AM Breakfast, 9-10AM a healthy snack like a piece of fruit, 12-1PM lunch, 2-3PM another healthy snack followed by dinner around 5-6PM.

A benefit of eating this way is that your metabolism will stay revved up because you are constantly digesting throughout the day (which burns calories). This also means your body is getting a continuous supply of nourishment and you can stay more active because you're not feeling weak or hungry. Likewise, you're not trying to make up for the longer gaps between meals by eating too much and getting stuck on the couch with a bloated belly!

Your metabolism will stay stronger when you eat the good stuff, like; whole grains, fresh fruits and veggies, while limiting or, better yet, eliminating processed foods. The reason for this is that it takes more work for your body to digest the good foods. This makes you feel full longer and you will burn more calories while digesting. Avoid eating "empty calories" because they do nothing for you. Don't forget your fluids too!

Spend a week counting your calories to get a better under-standing of what you're actually consuming. If you have a food item of which you're not sure how many calories it has, go to this website: (www.calorieking.com). You can type in the food item along with the size and it will tell you how many calories it contains. Corporations have done too great of a job with advertising telling us that eating larger sizes is the cool, 'manly' or good ol' American way to eat. You know why? Because as you get fatter, so do their bank accounts!

Remember, eat four to six times per day and spread your protein intake throughout the day to aid in tissue recovery. Consume your post workout meal within thirty to sixty minutes after your workout. Bare in mind this is only *basic* nutritional information. Seek the advice of an expert such as a Dietician or Certified Nutrition Consultant if you want to get more in depth and customize a plan for yourself.

Calculating Your Caloric Intake

Everything you consume can either positively or negatively affect your nutritional success. You now have learned that the types of food and the amount of food you consume each day are important. When working to change your body composition you need to know how many calories are enough or too much. Next you will find a chart by the *U.S. Department of Health and Human Services* to determine where you are calorie wise and how to adjust them to make the gains or losses you desire.

***The tables calculate the daily calories necessary to support your metabolic rate. Margin of error is +/- ten percent. To calculate your height in inches, just multiply the number of feet by twelve and then add the remainder of inches. So, for five foot five inches, the formula would be 5 x 12 = 60; then add the five inches, and you get sixty-five inches.

Note: If your goal is to lose weight, put in your ideal weight instead of your current weight to get an idea of how many calories to aim for. However, make sure to step down gradually so you don't shock your body into thinking something is wrong.

Men

1. Your Body Weight x 6.22   =   _____

2. Your Height (in inches) x 12.70   =   _____

   Now add both lines   +   _____66_____

   Subtotal   =   _____

3. Age (years) x 6.80   =   _____

   Then subtract the subtotal from this number.

   =   _____

   Caloric need to maintain current weight.

4. Activity Factor (from below)   _____

   x Caloric need above.

5. Total Daily Calories   =   _____

Women

1. Your Body Weight x 4.36   = _____

2. Your Height (in inches) x 4.32 = _____

    Now add both lines   + _____665_____

    Subtotal   = _____

3. Age (years) x 4.70   = _____

    Then subtract the
    subtotal from this
    number.

    = _____

    Caloric need to
    maintain current
    weight.

4. Activity Factor (from below)   _____

    x Caloric need above.

5. Total Daily Calories   = _____

Activity Factor

1.3 = Very light physical activity (sitting, driving, standing, lab work).

1.5 = Light physical activity (housecleaning, walking 3mph).

1.7 = Moderate physical activity (tennis, walking 4mph, weeding).

2.0 = Heavy physical activity (full court basketball, heavy digging, long distance running).

2.4 = Very heavy physical activity (competitive triathlete etc.)

If your goal is to lose weight, avoid lowering your caloric intake too much too soon. **It's very important to remember that a caloric deficit greater than five hundred to seven hundred calories on a daily basis will cause the body to actually slow down its metabolic rate and burn fewer calories.**

If you cut out too much too fast your body will go into survival mode and actually hold on to more of what you consume because it thinks something is wrong, and rightly so. It's not healthy for you to lose too much in a short period of time. Your body needs time to adjust and make changes. This is why fad diets that promise incredible weight losses don't work after a short period of time. Your body needs to be able to adjust to remain healthy. Keep in mind that it most likely took you years to put on the weight, which is why you really didn't notice it.

Remain safe with your goal by only lowering your calories by one hundred to two hundred per day. This will allow you to adjust properly and avoid "shocking" the body and causing a rebound. Not to mention it is much easier to do it this way. You won't feel like you're starving yourself as soon as you start – like with a lot of plans out there. For example, if you enjoy a large Caramel Frappuccino every day, all you would have to do is order a medium size instead. Simple right? By taking the baby-steps you're still going to enjoy the foods that you like instead of settling for a plate of carrots and rice cakes for a meal.

Note: It takes an extra 3,500 calories to put on 1-pound of fat. What this means is if you have stayed within you caloric range of, say two 2,500 calories for the day, but added two Mocha Espresso's to your diet each day, that's about an extra five hundred calories to your daily intake. At the end of the week you will have put on one-pound of fat (unless your burn it off).

Water

This is another topic that is always heated (no pun intended). How much water should you consume? Aside from staying hydrated, why exactly, is water so important? What if I drink a soda or coffee; does that count?

The Importance of Water

Water contributes to about sixty percent of the human body by weight. Although we can go a couple of *weeks* without food, we can only survive a few *days* without water. One important benefit of maintaining proper fluid balance is that fluid retention is *alleviated*. Yes, you read correctly. The human body has become so efficient that if it doesn't get enough water it will retain more of what you do consume to aid in survival. This is because the body doesn't know when the next supply will come. If you drink water regularly, it won't have a need to store as much. The same goes for food too. If you are overweight, increasing your water intake will help you dramatically because when you are feeling hungry, oftentimes you are actually thirsty. The body uses the same signals for hungry and thirsty and unfortunately most people get confused and feed themselves instead of drinking more water.

Other benefits of regular water consumption are:

✦ Liver function improves

✦ Natural thirst regulation returns

✦ Appetite decreases significantly

✦ Nutrients can be distributed throughout the body more efficiently

✦ Waste by-products are flushed from the body

How Water Affects Performance

Fluid loss of only two percent or more of your body weight will adversely affect circulatory function and decrease performance. Also, the body *cannot* adapt to dehydration. Just so you understand exactly what this means, here is the clinical definition of dehydration from WebMD:

Dehydration is often used in clinical practice to indicate the combined loss of both water and sodium. Many physiologists would have preferred the term to be used to indicate pure water loss. However, patients never lose only water.

Likewise, the term "re-hydration" is never used to mean giving patients pure water. Miscommunication between clinicians does not occur because detailed laboratory data such as serum

electrolytes, creatine, blood urea nitrogen and glucose levels as well as the type of fluids used to "re-hydrate" are always included in their conversation.

As we all know dehydration is not good for the body. Here is a list of the effects of dehydration.

+ Decrease in blood pressure
+ Decrease in sweat rate
+ Water retention
+ Increase in heart rate
+ Sodium (salt) retention
+ Decrease in blood flow to the skin
+ Increase in perceived exertion (feeling tired sooner)
+ Increase in muscle glycogen

Can You Have Too Much Water?

This may shock you but the answer is yes! Consuming too much water is called "water intoxication" or the technical term Hyponatremia. And it's not an unusual problem. Often seen in long-distance runners and cyclists, it can also be associated with obsessive-compulsive behaviors. Too much water in our system causes the dilution of essential electrolytes and sodium in our blood stream. What happens is that as the athlete consumes large amounts of water over the course of the event, blood plasma (the liquid part of blood) increases. As this takes place, the sodium content of the blood is diluted. At the same time, the athlete is losing sodium by sweating. Consequently, the amount of sodium available to body tissue will decrease over time to a point where the loss interferes with brain, heart, and muscle function.

How Much Should I Have?

We consume water in the form of liquids (juice, coffee etc.) and also in foods, primarily fruits and vegetables. The only foods that don't contain water are commercially dehydrated foods. Ideally you should drink approximately ninety-six ounces (or three quarts) each day. If your aim is weight loss, pay close attention to that last sentence. Water can curb your appetite and improve organ functions to aid greatly in your efforts.

As you exercise it's recommended that you consume sixteen ounces of fluids two hours before your workout. Drink twenty to forty ounces of fluids for every hour of exercise. If your workout is *more* than an hour at a time, drink a sports drink to replace electrolytes and muscle glycogen stores instead. If it is less than an hour, water will work best for you.

Basic Exercise Terms to Know

Knowing the basic terminology will, at the very least, give you more confidence in asking questions and advice from someone more experienced.

When I was in the Air Force, my training instructor would always say that the dumbest question you could ever ask is the one *you don't ask*. Nevertheless, all of us like to keep our pride in check and if you don't know what or how to ask the question you want, you'll never ask it for fear of looking foolish. Knowledge is power so; to set you minds at ease, I'll explain some basic terms to give you a nice boost.

I remember one time when I was teaching a workshop, a member asked the question "What *is* fitness? What exactly does it mean to be fit?" I thought this was a fantastic question. We hear about fitness all the time but very few of us take the time to ask ourselves "What would it take to consider myself fit?" If you're involved in sports or you look lean or muscular it would seem an easy answer but does *looking* fit mean that you *are* fit? What about the everyday person looking to achieve fitness? After I pondered this question for a while, this is what I came up with as the definition of "being fit" for the average person:

Being fit is the ability to handle everyday tasks and demands placed on the body with relative ease.

What this means is: are you able to climb a flight of stairs without being winded at the top? Can you pick up your kids or play with them without getting dizzy or "pooped" after only a few minutes? Can you carry bags of groceries from the car to the kitchen without having to stop to give your muscles a rest? If you can say yes to these questions, then I would venture it's safe to say you're in relatively good shape. Congratulations! With that said, here are some common terms that everyone needs to know when exercising:

Repetition or Rep – This is defined as one complete movement of a particular exercise involving the three muscle actions – concentric, isometric and eccentric (I'll explain what these are very shortly). Reps are simply a means to count the number of movements performed or a means to count how many times a particular muscle has been under tension.

How many reps you perform will depend on what your goal is. Research demonstrates that training in a specific repetition range yields specific benefits. Here is a table for a repetition range as offered by the *National Academy of Sports Medicine* (NASM):

Training Goal	Repetition Range
Beginners learning proper movement:	1-5
Building strength:	6-8
Building size (bodybuilding):	8-12
Developing muscle endurance:	12-25

The reason there is a repetition range and not a set number is because you need to properly fatigue the muscle in order to gain the benefits of your effort. Using bodybuilding as an example, the weight should be set to a point that you can no longer perform a complete rep while maintaining correct form between eight and twelve reps. If you are able to get to twelve reps or more while maintaining correct form, then increase the weight to the point where you reach the failure point between eight to twelve reps. If by adjusting the weight you can only get to, say, seven reps, then stay with that weight until you can reach twelve reps, then increase the weight again. If you are not *consistently* challenging your muscles you're not gong to achieve the results you are looking for. You'll only be wasting your time going through the motions.

Set or Sets – A set is a group of consecutive repetitions. For example, you may do three sets of eight repetitions. Just like the repetitions, the numbers of sets you perform are tailored to your goal. Here's a table outlining the suggested set range:

Training Goal	Set Range
Beginners learning proper movement:	4-8
Building strength:	3-4
Building size:	3
Developing muscle endurance:	1-3

Resting Periods

This is very important because it can have a dramatic affect on the outcome of your training. The resting period is the time taken to recuperate between sets. The ability to replenish energy supplies between sets is crucial for optimal performance while training.

By adjusting the rest period, energy supplies can be regained according to your goal. This is especially important for athletes training for sports.

20-30 seconds rest = approximately 50 percent recovery

40 seconds rest = approximately 75 percent recovery

60 seconds rest = approximately 85-90 percent recovery

3 minutes rest = approximately 100 percent recovery

The more rest you have between sets equals more energy for the next set. If you are an endurance athlete then you will want to train yourself to perform on less energy.

Motions of the Repetition

When you perform a repetition correctly there are actually three separate motions you are executing: the concentric, isometric and the eccentric. You may not hear these terms very often, but it's important to know what they are because there is quite a bit of reading material that will refer to these terminologies.

The **concentric** motion refers to when the muscle is contracted or flexed. Using a shoulder press as an example: the concentric motion is when you press your arms over your head. This is where you build most of your explosive power.

The **isometric** motion refers to the point when the muscle is fully contracted and you pause for a brief period stabilizing the joint. This can be anywhere from one to five seconds. This motion is an important part of the repetition because this is where you build joint stabilization by strengthening the smaller muscles that support the joint. Most people overlook this part of the rep and quickly press up and down only.

The **eccentric** motion refers to when you disengage the contraction of the muscle and move back to the starting point of the rep. It's commonly called the "negative". This is where you build the majority of your strength.

Note: True strength is not how much weight you can lift but rather how much weight you are able to control during the repetition.

Repetition Tempo

This I feel is a very important feature of the rep that I believe many trainers overlook. It refers to the speed in which you perform each rep. The speed in which you perform the rep can be manipulated to achieve specific goals.

Training Goal	Motions = Concentric-Isometric-Eccentric
Beginners learning proper movement: As fast as **safely** possible	1-1-1 seconds
Building Strength: Moderate speed	1-1-3 seconds
Building size (body building): Slow speed	2-2-4 seconds
Developing muscle endurance: Slow to moderate	1-2-1 seconds or 1-1-1 seconds

Resistance Training

Resistance training is simply working with weight that creates a resistance for a muscle to overcome or control. This can be your body weight, free weights, tubing, cables or machines. Many who exercise to lose weight believe that spending extended periods of time on cardio equipment is the best route to burn calories. However, this is not entirely true. Although you may feel like you're doing more for yourself because you are hot and dripping with sweat – and your *are* burning calories –, the most effective way to get rid of unwanted calories is resistance training, and your best path for a calorie-burning program is resistance training *supplemented* with cardiovascular training.

Here's why…

As your muscles develop and become more efficient they will have the need for more fuel. This revs your metabolism into high gear and your muscles will continue to burn stored energy (calories) even when you're not exercising!

Or to put it another way: cardio will increase your metabolism and keep it going for about thirty to forty *minutes* after you've finished exercising, while resistance training will increase your metabolism and keep it going for about three to four *hours* after you've finished!

Read that one again.

If you have religiously done cardio training to burn calories let it sink in before you move on.

Other benefits from resistance training are:

- ✦ Cardiovascular efficiency (helps strengthen the heart)
- ✦ Increased lean muscle mass (reduces body fat)
- ✦ Metabolic efficiency (burn calories longer)
- ✦ Increased tissue tensile strength (keeps muscles, tendon & ligaments from tearing)
- ✦ Increased bone density (less chance for osteoporosis or broken bones)
- ✦ Increase joint stability (reduced injuries)

A Woman's Fear

One of the constant obstacles for a trainer to overcome when introducing women to resistance training is that they are afraid of getting big or "buffed". Ladies, let me set your minds at ease: **it-is-very-hard-for-a-man-to-gain-muscle-mass** (without drugs). **It-is-ten-times-tougher-for-a-woman**. Now genetics *can* play a role but, for the most part, you have nothing to worry about. It takes a *very* dedicated lifestyle or enhancement drugs to get the kind of muscular physiques you see in body building shows and magazines. Even popular movie stars have to dedicate time with a personal trainer and a nutritionist to obtain their physiques. And yes, some of them use steroids or other enhancement drugs too.

Ninety-nine percent of all women that I have trained want to lose weight as their exercise goal. Let me explain to you – and this goes for the guys too - if you want to lose weight fast, keep it off, and make it last, resistance training is the most powerful weapon for you to accomplish this with.

With that said, let's go into some choices in routines. The two most common exercise routines available for you are the **Split Routine** and **Circuit Training**.

Split Routine

The split routine has been around since the early years of weightlifting. This is a routine that separates the body into parts to be trained on separate days. Training this way allows you to really focus on the muscle group that you're exercising and allows for adequate time for each muscle group to rest and recuperate.

There are several theories in regards to how often you should let each muscle group rest before you exercise them again. The resting period can range anywhere from three to ten days.

However, it's widely accepted that it takes about five days for a muscle to fully recuperate.

I've had great success with a seven-day split routine. My workouts are fairly short and I don't feel tired throughout the week. Here's an example of how it works:

Each muscle group is exercised once every seven days and you can mix the groups up any way you prefer. I generally recommend starting with the larger muscle groups at the beginning of the week when you have the most energy.

Monday –   Quadriceps & Hamstrings

Tuesday –   Back

Wednesday –   Rest Day

Thursday –   Chest & Shoulders

Friday –   Core & Calves

Saturday –   Biceps & Triceps

Sunday –   Rest Day

Here is what a ten-day split routine looks like. Each muscle group is exercised every ten days.

Monday –   Quadriceps & Hamstrings

Tuesday –   Rest Day

Wednesday –   Back

Thursday –   Chest

Friday –   Rest Day

Saturday –   Shoulders & Calves

Sunday –   Core

Monday –   Biceps

Tuesday –   Triceps

Wednesday –   Rest Day

Thursday –   Start again with Quadriceps & Hamstrings

The ten-day split allows for a lot of recuperation and it allows you to *really* focus on each muscle group. This is a good routine if you have a busy schedule as it allows for more days off during the week. Find what works best for you and have fun with it.

Circuit Routine

This routine involves performing a series of exercises in succession with minimal rest. This typically involves one to three sets (usually only one or two) of twelve to twenty repetitions with only ten to forty seconds rest in between each set. These variables, however, can be changed to achieve the desired outcome. The two most common circuit routines involve either exercising all muscle groups per workout or alternating the body into upper and lower halves per workout.

This has been a great routine for those who are short on time or those who don't have a set schedule they can adhere to each week. The idea is to make the most out of your time and not neglect any part of your body.

Here is a sample of a circuit routine, performing one to two sets per muscle group with cardio five days of the week:

Monday –   Routine plus Cardio

Tuesday –   Cardio Only

Wednesday –   Routine plus Cardio

Thursday –   Cardio Only

Friday –   Routine plus Cardio

Saturday –   Rest Day

Sunday -   Rest Day

Here is what a split circuit routine looks like:

Monday –   Upper Body plus Cardio

Tuesday –   Lower Body plus Cardio

Wednesday –   Cardio Only

Thursday –   Upper Body plus Cardio

Friday –   Lower Body plus Cardio

Saturday –   Rest Day

Sunday -   Rest Day

Again, you can mix this up to fit your needs or schedule. As you can see I've added cardio five days a week, however, you can add cardio up to six days per week or every other day if you like. I'll touch more on cardio later. However, you'll want to give yourself at least two days off back-to-back per week in order to rest and recuperate.

As a reminder you can perform one to three sets with this routine. I've had some clients who like to do one set for each body part as they go through the whole circuit and then do the circuit again if they have time or, they may do two sets per body part as they go through the circuit. These are only two of the most commonly used training routines and will be sufficient to get you started. However, if you're the type who likes more options in life, here is a list of other routines you can try.

More Routines

Single-Set Routine

Performing only one set *per exercise* and not to be confused with the circuit routine where you perform one set per *body part.* For example, you might complete one set of bench press and one set of incline bench press.

Multiple-Set Routine

As the name implies, this is performing multiple sets per exercise. This is most often done with the split-routine. For example: three sets of bench press, three sets of incline press and three sets of pectoral flies.

Super-Set Routine

Performing two different exercises in rapid succession with no rest in between. For example, doing a set of arm curls and then immediately followed by a set of triceps extensions. Or standing curls immediately followed by preacher curls.

Pyramid Routine

This has each set progressing up or down in weight. For example, your first set may start with ten pounds, then your second set with twenty pounds, your third with thirty pounds and so on. You can also reverse this starting with thirty pounds and moving down to ten pounds.

If your goal is bodybuilding this is a great routine as you will be able to stay within you repetition range but continually challenge the muscle being worked.

Oxygen

Oxygen is the necessary catalyst for many of the body's functions when engaged in continuous activity for thirty minutes or longer. Here are two important terms you need to know:

Aerobic – pronounced (air·o·bic)

When you're involved in extended cardiovascular activity, it is called aerobic. Meaning it requires oxygen to complete the task. Running on a treadmill is an example of an aerobic activity.

Anaerobic – Pronounced (an·air·o·bic)

This is the term for activities that last for short durations and are not dependent on oxygen for completion. Resistance training is an example of an anaerobic activity.

Note: Even though resistance training is anaerobic you still need to breathe. I catch people all the time holding their breath when lifting. This can cause you to get light-headed, dizzy and produce headaches.

The Cardio-Respiratory Systems

Cardio is the abbreviated term given to cardiovascular activities. This is exercise that places stress on the cardio-respiratory system (aerobic). These activities can be anything from walking, biking, running to swimming, basketball, soccer and so forth.

The *cardio-respiratory* system is an abbreviation for two systems: the cardiovascular system and the respiratory system. Because they work hand-in-hand, the two terms are often combined. Together they provide the body with oxygen, nutrients, protective agents and a way to remove waste by-products. I want to separate and explain each part of the cardio-respiratory system so you can have a better understanding of why cardio activities are important to include in your exercise program.

The Cardiovascular System

This system is an accumulation of the heart, the blood it pumps, the blood vessels and arteries that transports the blood from the heart to the rest of the body. Your body utilizes this system to gather the necessary oxygen and nutrients for daily function and repairs.

The Respiratory System

The primary role of this system is to ensure proper cellular functioning. The respiratory system accomplishes this by providing a means to collect oxygen from the environment by breathing in and transport the oxygen to the bloodstream to be circulated where needed.

Cardio Training

First let me start by informing you why it is important to have cardio training as part of your overall exercise program. The heart moves blood to the lungs, where the blood picks up oxygen; the blood then brings the oxygen to the muscles, which utilize the oxygen along with nutrients as fuel. The used oxygen is then routed back to the lungs to start the process all over again, while the blood removes the waste by-products from the muscles.

The body needs more oxygen with increased intensity levels, thus making the heart work more to pump oxygen-rich blood to the muscles. As your fitness level increases and your heart becomes stronger, it will be able to pump more blood with every beat. As a result, your heart won't have to beat as often to get the needed oxygen and nutrients to your muscles. This will decrease your resting heart rate and your exercising heart rate on all exertion levels. Simply put, this means you won't get "winded" so quickly and you will be able to recover from intense exercise more rapidly.

Now let's cover the different aspects of cardio training. Unless you've been instructed on the importance of taking the time to warm up and cool down it's easily, and more often than not, a much neglected or improperly performed portion of your workout. However, the benefits of the warm-up and the cool-down are numerous.

There are two components that you should include into your warm-up and cool-down.

1. **Aerobic Activity** – This can be almost anything you enjoy such as walking, biking, running, using the elliptical trainer, or playing a game of racquetball. Just make sure to perform your activity with gradual intensity to reduce the risk of injury.

2. **Stretching** – There are three distinct stretching methods.

    ✦ **Self-myofascial release** (SMR) - This is commonly called 'foam roll stretching' and is best performed *before* the aerobic portion of the warm up.

    ✦ **Static stretching** is the most common way to stretch. This is the stretch that you hold for several seconds and should only be done *after* you are finished exercising.

    ✦ **Active stretching** should be done in place of static stretching and is the best way to stretch *before* a sporting event.

You'll learn more about stretching later.

The Warm-Up

The purpose of the warm-up is to get your body prepared to exercise. The warm-up does this by gradually increasing your heart rate, blood pressure, and oxygen consumption to performance levels. This is combined with the dilation of blood vessels, and increased heat produced by the working muscles that help to increase their elasticity.

Think of your muscles, ligaments and tendons as rubber bands. If you put a rubber band in the freezer for a while and take it out, what happens when you try to stretch it? It snaps in half. Likewise, if you lay the rubber band on a hot sidewalk on a sunny day and then try to stretch it – it stretches far beyond what you thought was possible. Your muscles act in the same way.

The big question I get all the time about the warm-up is: 'How long should it be?' Well, it's generally accepted to be a *minimum* of ten minutes and sometimes longer in the winter months when you feel chilled to the bone.

Note: You are not only warming up your muscles, but also your ligaments and tendons. Ligaments and tendons have poor blood-flow compared to muscles and need this time to warm up properly. Don't only go by how your muscles feel.

The Cool-Down

This is a portion that is notoriously overlooked – even by a lot of trainers I've worked with. The cool-down is vitally important for just as many reasons as the warm-up. It ensures that there will be adequate circulation to the muscles, heart, and brain by preventing any sudden blood 'pooling' in the muscles. As you now know, your muscles fill up with blood to provide them with the necessary oxygen and nutrients to perform the given task when you are involved with any kind of exercise. Likewise, the blood flushes out the waste by-products to make room for the fresh replacements of nutrients and oxygen. Thus the cool-down can aid in preventing and reducing the likelihood of such things as dizziness, fainting, and the development of sore muscles caused by waste by-products not being properly flushed out of the muscles.

I'm sure everyone has experienced the latter. All the elements that the cool-down helps prevent are reasons a lot of well-meaning beginners tend to quit. Extensive research has shown the direct association between properly and consistently performing the warm-up and cool-down with improvements in overall performance and achieving fitness goals, as well as, the reduction in the risk of injury. Now we'll discuss the two types of cardio training.

Cardio Guidelines

According to NASM cardio training means any type of physical activity that involves and places stress on your cardiorespiratory system. There are three aspects of your cardio training that you should consider when setting up a cardio program:

Frequency: To maintain general health the recommended frequency if preferably everyday for about twenty to thirty minutes (or what you are capable of doing). However, when you are just starting out and are looking to improve you fitness levels, the frequency should be about three to five days per week.

Intensity: For general health maintenance your cardio exercise should be at a moderate intensity to make sure you are placing enough demand on your system but not necessarily bringing your self to exhaustion or breathlessness. To improve your fitness levels I would recommend that you exercise within sixty to eighty-five percent of your maximum heart rate.

Time: What has been learned about cardio training is that it doesn't have to be completed all at one time. For example: if your goal is to include thirty minutes of cardio a day you can break it up and complete ten minutes in the morning, ten minutes in the afternoon, and ten minutes in the evening. Likewise, if you spend an hour at the health club, you could complete ten minutes then move on to complete a few sets of your resistance training then come back and complete another ten minutes of your cardio training and so forth. For some, this helps to break up their routine and keeps it interesting.

How Does Monitoring Your Heart Rate (HR) Work?

It has become more mainstream in recent years to train in your target heart rate zone. By doing so, you will achieve goals faster. Here are some reasons why:

Having direct measurement of your HR during exercise is the most accurate way to judge your performance. This aids in keeping you from over-training or under-training. As a benefit your progress can be monitored and measured, increasing your motivation.

Monitoring you HR can help maximize your benefits if you have a limited amount of time to exercise. These days most machines have built-in HR programs that will have the machine (treadmill, elliptical etc.) adjust itself if you're wearing a heart rate monitor, and keep you in your targeted heart rate zone. This is great for those who like to read or watch TV while doing cardio.

Here's the formula to calculate your heart rate training zones:

220 – Your Age x 0.8 = 80 percent of your maximum heart rate.

220 – Your Age x 0.6 = 60 percent of your maximum heart rate.

There is a variety of HR monitors out today. Shop around for one that suits you and your budget. One brand that I recommend is *Polar*®. They have been in business for a long time and have a solid track record for quality. They also will work with almost all top-name cardio machines around today.

Flexibility Training

Stretching is one of those things that seem to be a side thought with exercise programs. Rarely do I come across someone who is putting real focus on this part of the workout. Flexibility training has many benefits, like for example, decreasing the chance for muscle imbalances or even correcting the imbalances that pull your posture out of correct alignment.

Muscle imbalances are an alteration in the length of the muscle surrounding a joint. Meaning some muscles are shortened or tight on one side of the joint while others may be lengthened on the opposite side thus limiting or altering correct movement. It's really impossible to have proper function and performance without proper flexibility. Limited flexibility decreases your body's adaptive potential by forcing it to move in *altered* movements. Almost everyone has altered movement to some degree and may not even be aware of it because the altered pattern has been the 'normal' movement for some time.

Cumulative Injury Cycle

Poor posture, repetitive movements and injuries can create a dysfunction within the connective tissue surrounding a joint. The body treats this dysfunction as an injury in which it will then initiate a repair process. Tennis Elbow is a common cumulative injury. I don't want to confuse you with the lengthy details, so to see if this is something you have, get some input from a qualified trainer or, visit your Chiropractor or medical practitioner.

Definition of Flexibility

So what is flexibility? Flexibility is "the normal extensibility of all soft tissues that allow the full range of motion of a joint".

Types of Stretching

As mentioned earlier, there are three types of stretching methods you can use with your exercise program.

1. **Static Stretching** – This is most likely the type of stretching that you are familiar with. This involves passively taking a muscle to the point of tension and holding the stretch for about twenty to thirty seconds without "bouncing". This style of stretching combines low force with long duration movements. This allows the soft tissue to relax and provide for better elongation. An example would be to bend over to touch your toes and holding yourself in that position for twenty to thirty seconds.

Note: This should only be done *after* your workout or sport. The reason is that this type of stretching can decrease muscle strength by up to twenty percent, which can last up to thirty minutes.

2. **Active Stretching** – This is the recommended way to stretch before a workout or sport. This type of stretching allows for greater range of motion to be accessed and moves the muscle that closely mimics the movements you are about to do for your workout.

    With golfing, for example, this type of stretching would involve swinging the club loosely back and forth for about twenty to thirty seconds or laying the club across your shoulders and twisting back and forth.

3. **Self-Myofascial Release** (SMR) – Have you ever seen those white foam rolls that are four feet long at the health club? This is what they're for. This is more commonly called foam roll stretching. SMR is another form of flexibility training that focuses on the fascia system in the muscle. This involves applying gentle force to the muscle to release the 'knots' in the muscle fibers and bring them back into alignment, allowing them to function properly. A good massage will do the same thing. Ask a personal trainer to show you how to do this correctly.

I hope that I've clarified how important flexibility training is to your overall routine. Sometimes I will take a client and work with them for two weeks just on stretching and cardio alone in order to get the muscles, or more accurately the joints, to function properly before we begin any resistance training. Otherwise, if we moved right into the resistance portion and the client has obvious postural imbalances, I may further increase those imbalances, worsening their effect and/or creating a cumulative injury cycle.

Your Posture

Having and maintaining proper posture is very important. I'm not talking about being able to walk across a room with a book on your head but of having your spine and joints aligned properly. How you carry yourself through your posture helps determine how well your muscles and joints work, how well your organs function, how smoothly your nerves, blood vessels and your lymph passages work and how strong your bones are.

Because your posture has more to it than just sitting up straight, it affects every single part of your body. If you spend the majority of your day sitting, whether it's for work or pleasure, chances are that your posture is causing you a great deal of harm – and you may not realize it yet.

The main factors that cause postural imbalances include:

✦ Postural stress (slouching for extended periods)

✦ Repetition of movement or pattern overload (performing tasks in bad posture)

✦ Lack of movement (lazy butts on the couch all day – uh huh, be honest)

And injuries that will cause you to alter your movement pattern to the point they become 'normal' movements (like having a sprained ankle).

Not only will proper posture improve your muscle and nerve function but it will improve your flexibility as well. To give you an example: grab a chair and a broomstick and sit in front of a mirror if you can, or get a partner to observe you. Hold the broomstick across your shoulders either in front or behind your head; now, in your normal, slouched sitting position (no cheating), twist as far as you safely can. Take note on how far the end of the broom goes.

Ok, now sit up straight with proper posture. Again twist to one side. You should notice that you were able to twist further to the side than when you were slouched. If you didn't notice any change, well, we need to work on your flexibility!

Nonetheless, even if you noticed only a small change, this will improve as you continue your exercise program. My point with this demonstration is how much safer proper posture is just in flexibility. If you were, say, snow skiing and took a tumble, just by being able to twist that little bit more could mean the difference from laughing it off or being sledded down the mountain by the rescue team. Even in every-day-life, like picking boxes off the ground to put on a shelf, having that little extra could keep you from having to spend the day lying on the couch in pain.

Neutral Spine

This is a term you will hear more often as you evolve in your fitness experience, especially if you work with a trainer. If you were to look at your spine from the side you'd notice the spine has a natural 'S' curve to it.

Neutral spine refers to positioning yourself, whether you're sitting or standing, with your spine in its natural position. It's in the optimal position to allow an equal distribution of force throughout the entire body.

In neutral posture, the body is able to function in its strongest, most balanced position. Stress to the joints, muscles, vertebrae and tissue is minimized. Maintaining neutral posture will help decrease the risk of injury and increase the efficiency of movement.

When people have difficulty achieving or working in neutral posture, it is often an indication of muscular imbalance. Muscular or postural imbalances are a concern because they can lead to injury, chronic injuries or limit performance. Working out of neutral alignment may inhibit the recruitment of certain muscles and make the movements more difficult.

Here's how to achieve neutral spine:

1. Place your feet hip-width apart (this is closer together than shoulder distance apart, which is a common position).

2. Begin by straightening up into a full standing position with your hands on your hips. The knees should remain softened, not locked.

3. Focus on finding the neutral position of the pelvis by rotating your hips backwards to the furthest point and then rotate your hips forward to the furthest point.

    What you want is the middle (neutral) position. You may have to keep rotating your hips forward and backwards in increasingly smaller motions until you get it. Your belt-line should be horizontal and not tilting forward or backwards.

4. Now take you hands off your hips and relax your shoulders down and roll them back. You should be able to draw a straight line from the center of one shoulder across to the center of the other. Think about bringing your shoulder blades in towards your spine. They should rest flat on you back.

5. Bring your head into alignment by centering your ears over your shoulders. You might need to extend your chin forward or back to find the centered position. Have a partner help guide you into position and if possible have them take a picture of you before and after so you can see the difference for yourself.

6. Review the natural position of the spine. Feel the feet centering the weight of the body and solidly supporting you on the floor. You should feel ready to move in any

direction. You can also have your partner safely press down on your shoulders in both positions so you can feel the difference of pressure on your spine.

This position will require work to maintain. Even though it is supposed to be the natural alignment of the body, most people have developed habits and imbalances that make it feel unnatural. However, it is essential to strengthen the muscles into proper alignment, and establishing neutral posture is the first step. Try to increase your awareness of neutral posture in your daily activities. Better yet: have a chiropractor or personal trainer to help you with this. Remember all those times your mother told you to stand up straight? All these years you were getting excellent fitness advice!

"Locking-Out" Joints

Locking out a joint is a common term that refers to straightening the joint until it 'locks' into an unready position. Some may even brag about being "double-jointed", bending a joint past its natural position. This is a bad place to be in. Not only are you placing undue stress and wear-and-tear on the joint but you are learning bad postural habits as well.

You may notice when you begin a movement you have to unlock the joint before you begin. By locking-out the knee joints you can dramatically reduce the blood flow to the brain, and cause you to get light-headed or even pass out. In short, I ask that you *never* lockout your joints. It may take some conscious thinking and practice but you'll be better off for it.

Your Work Environment

As many of you have desk jobs these days, make an effort to practice good posture. If your employer will allow you, replace your chair with a stability ball or put a note up where you can see it to remind you to reposition yourself. As well as sitting up straight, make sure to pull your belly button in toward your spine. This strengthens the Transversus Abdominis, which is an important abdominal muscle. A weakened Transversus Abdominis is the major culprit to chronic low back pain. Sitting at a desk all day easily weakens it. You may find that the aches and pains that have plagued your back will disappear in a short while if you practice pulling your belly button in with *any* activity.

Slouching during a long commute can cause aches, which, combined with slouching at your desk (and possibly the couch) all day will make you grumpy and tired and unmotivated to do anything else. In fact, when in your car, you can strengthen your abs by pulling your belly button in and pressing your lower back into the seat. Try to keep it up as long as you can.

The Core

What is the Core?

As little back as ten years ago a common phrase was "Tighten the abs, gotta have strong abs". Everything was about abdominal strength and flat bellies. But, as we learn more about the body, nowadays it's all about the core.

The core is a group of muscles that stabilize your mid-section. These are: the Transversus Abdominis, Internal Oblique, Multifidi, Pelvic Floor Muscles, the Diaphragm and the Thoratic and Cervical part of the spine.

Note: I purposely gave you the actual names of the muscle so you can look them up and see where they are.

The core is the center of the body and it is where *most* movement begins.

The core must be strong not only for exercise but for everyday movements. Efficient movement requires dynamic postural control, appropriate muscular balance and joint motion throughout the core. To achieve proper stabilization strength for the core, you must place the body in *controlled* unstable environments that requires balance, hence the stability ball.

Stability balls, even though an Italian engineer created them, are also call Swiss balls as they were used extensively in Switzerland back in the sixties for physical therapy. An example exercise would be a stability ball crunch. With this exercise you will need core stabilization to maintain spine stabilization, as well as neuromuscular stabilization control to stay balanced.

A core stabilization-training program will help you gain strength, neuromuscular control (this is the improvement of the nervous system's communication with the muscular system), power, and muscular endurance. If you are trying to lose weight, incorporating a stability program will help greatly too.

With a stability program, instead of exercising only the larger main muscle groups, you will involve all the smaller muscle groups that support a joint to perform the same movement. The more muscles involved – the more calories you'll burn! Not to mention these exercises are more reflective of real-world movements. You will also gain strength when you include these smaller muscle groups.

As time goes on we discover more about how the body functions. In recent years something we have learned is that performing only traditional abdominal exercises without proper internal pelvic stabilization has been shown to increase pressure on the vertebrae discs and compressive forces on the spine. Likewise, only performing traditional low back exercises without proper internal abdominal stabilization has been shown to increase pressure on the discs to dangerous levels, even causing damage to the ligaments supporting the vertebrae and leading to the narrowing of the openings in the vertebrae that the spinal nerves pass through. Needless to say, that's pretty scary stuff. And the thing is we may not know the full effects of training this way until years down the road.

Now that we covered the importance of the core, we can touch on the abs alone. You'll want to tighten your abs before you begin a movement in order to stabilize the spine. I've found over the years that, because we have several abdominal muscles, most people aren't sure of which muscles to tighten. However, now that you know your core, here's how to pull your belly button in to get stabilized and be ready for action.

The Drawing-in Maneuver

Begin by getting into neutral spine position. Once that's accomplished…

1. Take a deep breath using the diaphragm (not expanding the ribs). If your shoulders rise up it means you're expanding your ribs to take in air and not your diaphragm. You will learn more on breathing soon.

2. Now exhale while simultaneously pulling the navel in towards the spine and away from your clothing. Remember to stay in neutral spine position while doing

this. Do this without looking like you have sucked in your stomach. Sometimes it helps to place your hand just below the navel. The whole area should become flattened not 'caved in'.

3. Now keep this abdominal position and continue normal breathing. There should only be slight movement as your diaphragm moves. Remember, as you develop your cardio system, you will be able to take in more oxygen this way so don't get discouraged if this seems hard to do now.

4. You should hold this position as best as you can while performing any exercises or every day movements.

If you need to perform your reps slowly in order to keep your abdominal drawn in and stay in neutral spine, that's fine. Practice makes perfect and soon you won't have to think about it.

Breathing

Breathing During Reps

Some of you may be reading this and think, "Hey, I know how to breathe. I've been doing it all my life". However, there's more to breathing than you think. For example, there are two ways we get oxygen into our lungs:

1. By using the muscles within the ribs to expand the ribcage, along with other muscles such as the Scalenes, Sternocleidomastiod, Levator Scapulae and the Upper Trapezius. With breathing, these are considered secondary muscles. Breathing from the secondary muscles is more noticeable when we're "winded" and need more oxygen.

2. The other and preferred way is by using our diaphragm to pull air into our lungs. This is our normal way to breathe and it's how we get the most oxygen into our lungs. This is why you always hear of vocal coaches preaching, "Breathe from the diaphragm".

One thing that I've found with a majority of new clients is they hold their breath or breathe backwards. Huh, breathe backwards? What I mean is this: when you are performing a repetition there is a cadence to your breathing. Contrary to what a lot of people do, you want to breathe out when you contract the muscle.

Remember, this is the power (concentric) part of the rep. When you release the muscle contraction (eccentric) and go back to the beginning of the movement this is the time to breathe in. Never hold your breath as this can cause you to get light-headed or even pass out.

Dysfunctional Breathing

Breathing from the secondary muscles as mentioned before can become habitual. Breathing like this while exercising can cause excessive tension, which often results in headaches, lightheadedness and dizziness. If this is something you have experienced, incorrect breathing may be the culprit.

Also, excessive breathing – short shallow breaths - can lead to altered carbon dioxide and oxygen blood content that can lead to feelings of anxiety, which will further initiate excessive breathing. This can activity in pain receptors, creating increases in pain, retention of waste by-products within the muscle that can cause fatigue, as well as stiff and sore muscles.

As I mentioned before, there is a more to breathing than meets the eye. Don't let this discourage you though. If you have to practice proper breathing, the learning curve is very short. It soon takes over and becomes something you just do subconsciously.

Basic Movements You Should Know

As every exercise will have its own description for proper execution, my goal here is to give you some essentials for the most basic of movements that you will make so you can build a good foundation for your exercises. Again, as a reminder, before you begin any exercise make sure your posture is correct from head-to-toe and pull your belly button in (notice a pattern yet?).

General Upper Body Presses

During most pressing exercises you'll want to make sure that your wrist stays aligned or centered over your elbow. This is where your power and support is. Also, make sure that your wrist is straight and not bent forward or backwards compared to your arm. This is called neutral wrist. If, when holding a dumbbell or barbell, you bring your wrist out of the neutral position you can create a potential injury. Be aware, there are some bodybuilding techniques that claim that bringing the wrist out of its neutral position will yield better results with certain exercises this however, is not a good idea for the majority of exercises.

Next, when performing any pressing motions be sure you stop before your elbows are fully extended or locked-out as we discussed before. Keep the joint "soft" as it's called. During the eccentric (or negative) part of the press it's a good rule of thumb to stop when your elbow forms a ninety-degree angle.

It is a very common misconception when lifting (especially in bodybuilding) to bring a muscle to a 'deep stretch' with each rep. As we've discussed with static stretching: going to a deep stretch during a repetition confuses the muscle on your intensions - stretch or contract - and, as we have discussed already, it can reduce your strength for up to thirty minutes. It is much better to keep the muscle engaged throughout the complete repetition. When performing the chest press or something similar, if you go too far past the ninety-degree angle in your elbow you will *disengage* the pectoral muscle (chest) and stretch it across the rib cage, which takes it out of the exercise and forces the front deltoid (shoulder) and triceps to handle the load.

If you have ever done a bench-press before then most likely you know about that point in the rep where you hit a pause a few inches above the chest; and sometimes you have to have your spotter bump you up a bit; this is because the pectorals are not engaged. As soon as they do engage, you can push the bar the rest of the way yourself.

It is much better to stop at the ninety-degree angle than to bring the bar all the way to the chest. This is a power lifting technique and is not beneficial for anyone else. By utilizing the ninety-degree angle you will see superior results, especially if your goal is bodybuilding or strength. You will also dramatically reduce your chances for injuries.

General Lower Body Presses

For the lower body presses you'll follow the same rule of thumb in motion mentioned for the upper-body presses regarding the ninety-degree angle and the locking-out of the joints. In the past I've come across health club members that don't like to do lower body presses like the squat. The most common reason is because it hurts their knees or lower back. Usually I'll take them aside for five or ten minutes, go over a few tips and presto, they're believers again! The biggest predicament I find is that they forget about posture. What many may not realize is that if you position your lower-body in a bad posture positions, it not only will affect the joints of your legs but your back as well.

So when performing lower-body exercises make sure that you start in the correct position and stay there. Pull the belly button in and have your feet facing forward. Your knees should be aligned with your middle toe. With squats, your toes can point slightly outward for comfort.If you feel forced to pull your knees inward or outward because of bad postural habits or because of excessive body weight, try to get into the proper position as much as possible.

Note: It may even be more beneficial to use smaller movements instead so you don't compromise proper form. Use a mirror to monitor your movements for better results.

Lower body presses are important to include with your program because they are very beneficial. For guys, even though we want the bulging pecs and biceps, it looks silly to have a well-developed upper body but have really skinny legs. Most women will agree.

Likewise, almost all women I've trained want toned thighs, hips and butts. Lower body presses like squats and lunges will incorporate all those muscle groups at once. This will save you time and give you the results you're looking for.

General Pulling Exercises

When you perform a pulling exercise, the target muscle group is mainly one back muscle or another. The biceps are secondary muscles that get involved after the target back muscle. However, I find most people use the biceps more than the intended back muscle. Therefore, when executing your pulling (or back) exercise, you should be made aware to concentrate on engaging the intended back muscle first, squeezing it as much as possible, and then include the biceps. This might be one of those times that you're thinking "Well duh", but this takes practice for most people. The biceps are muscles we use more frequently throughout the day and therefore subconsciously become the dominant muscles with these exercises.

Machines

Before we move on I wanted to touch-base on a key point whenever you use machines to exercise with at a health club. The thing I want you to remember is to make sure that the joint that is moving (elbow for curls, knee for leg extensions etc.) is lined up with the axis, or moving pivot, of the machine that you are using. When they are not lined up it can cause discomfort or possibly injury to your joint. Most machines in health clubs will have a red or black dot at the axis point to indicate where you should position your joint. Ask a trainer to help you spot these on the machines.

Setting Goals

In order to reach your goal, you have to first know what you want. Most know this already but the reality is this one simple step is almost always overlooked or done incorrectly even though it can be the most important step you take. And it's not good enough just to say, *"I want to lose weight"*. To really make it work you have to be specific (and realistic). For example:

"I want to lose ten percent of body fat in twelve weeks. In order to do this I'll need to lose 1.2 percent per week and I should only consume "X" amount of calories per day".

Then outline how you are going to do it. Meaning, how are you going to change your eating habits? How many times are you going to exercise per week? Are you going to have a personal trainer to help you?

Then write it down and sign it!

If you are married or have a significant other, have them sign it too. This gives your goal credibility, as well as making the commitment to your self. Over the years, my clients that did this and stood by it *always* achieved their goal. Read it out loud before you go to bed and when you wake up so it stays fresh in your mind. Do this with your spouse or partner too. Keep your goals alive in your mind all the time. A great way to grasp a hold on how to make and set goals is a book by Napoleon Hill called *The 17 Principals to Success*. It's a masterpiece for achieving *any* goal. I highly recommend it.

The Big Picture vs. The Next Step

A well-known proverb states, "A journey of a thousand miles begins with the first step". You should always keep the "big picture" in the back of your mind so you know what you are aiming for and when you've reached it. I find what works great for me is to focus my attention on the next step in front of me. This way I don't become overwhelmed looking at the goal in its entirety or with all that needs to take place.

Just take the first thing you want to accomplish and complete it, then move on to the next step and complete that. Not only does it feel more manageable but also you'll develop a continual sense of accomplishment, which feels great! This not only puts you in a positive frame of mind but also makes you eager to complete the next task. You can even purchase a fitness journal, make one yourself or get a software program that will help you track your progress. It soon gets to be exciting and fun to make and track your progress. It can become very addicting!

Last but not Least…

As the famous slogan says – **JUST DO IT!** So many clients talk themselves out of going to the gym or even begin their workout when they start to think about it too much. I'm guilty of this myself from time to time, especially when I'm tired from a long day at work.

The best thing to do is to put your mind on autopilot – have your gym clothes in your car and go straight from work to the gym. When you go home first, you can get comfortable and open too many chances to get sidetracked. The fact of the matter is, no matter how tired you are you *always* feel great after a workout! Not only does it improve your mood, you also don't have that nagging guilt from skipping out. Another mistake I find people make is they wait for the right time to start. Folks, there rarely is a 'perfect' time to start. If you continue the waiting game it's called PROCRASTINATION. Just start and everything else will soon fall into place.

Personal Trainers

The information that is compiled in this book is basic, general information. The human body is far too complex to be able to cover everything in one simple book. The fun is in the adventure when learning specialized details that will pertain to you and your particular goals. Like giving you the actual names of muscles that I've discussed. I did this so you can look them up and know exactly where they are and how they function – if you want to. My goal is to provide you with solid information to begin an exercise program with. However, if you decide you would like to work with a Personal Trainer at some point, here are a few suggestions to help you find a qualified person.

Qualifications

There are almost as many different training institutes issuing personal training certifications, as there are personal trainers. It happens that when I was starting out in getting my first certification it was with a very reputable organization. They get very in-depth with practical training methods. I remember when

I was studying for my test thinking, "Holy smokes, a trainer has to know all that"?

As I became more involved in the industry and learned who-was-who and what-was-what I was shocked to find out that there are companies that were offering a training certification in only two days (after all the studying that I did)! Others I found were a fraction of the cost or were only valid in certain cities or health clubs. However, when working alongside these other "trainers" I could spot a big difference. Now that personal training is accepted as a desired profession there are a good number of trainers that have a formal education connected to exercise like: Biomechanics and Kinesiology. However, when it comes to training certifications here are just some of the better certifications to look for:

- ✦ National Academy of Sports Medicine (NASM)
- ✦ American Council on Exercise (ACE)
- ✦ International Sports Sciences Association (ISSA)
- ✦ American College of Sports Medicine (ACSM)
- ✦ International Fitness Professionals Association (IFPA)
- ✦ International Sports Sciences Association (ISSA)

These are only *some* of the better certifications to look for and not necessarily in this order. If the trainer you're considering has a certification with one or more of the institutions above, it's a pretty good bet that they'll know what they are doing. Something to keep in mind however is that they each have a focus on different aspects of fitness. They each follow their own method of what they believe is the best approach to exercise. Do a little research to find out what each approach is about and which method seems the best match for your needs. You can do this by going to each company's website or sit down and chat with a trainer and let them explain it to you in their own words.

Experience

No matter what certification your trainer has, experience speaks volumes. Not only is experience important for the trainer to convert their newfound knowledge into practical use but it also teaches them how to communicate with clients. This communication is important and it's one aspect that many trainers seem to overlook (or learn the hard way). When a trainer goes through the training course to get certified' everything is taught in technical and medical terms. When working with clients the best trainers are the ones who can take these technical terms and convey them to their clients in layman's terms. I myself would go beyond telling my clients *what* to do and explain *why* they were being asked to do it. I would even give them pop quizzes to help them retain information. To me, this builds value in the tasks that I asked my clients to perform, which in turn gives them more motivation because sometimes the task may seem strange to them. It also makes the client feel like they are more of a part to the training process instead of being lead by the hand and told what to do somewhat like a child.

This was important for me to learn because, as adults, sometimes we feel vulnerable when we ask for help. This is a big deal for a lot of us to admit when it's a topic we may be uncomfortable with or self-conscious about already. I recommend finding a trainer who has about six to twelve months of experience under their belt. However, if you are hearing good things about someone who is newer, have a look and you may find a person that is very talented. Most trainers will have a short biography posted at the health club that highlights their experience and qualifications. Ask the front desk at your health club about where to find them.

Trainer Testimonials

Along with experience, ask around and see whom others recommend. Ask not only other club members but also the employees as they might have more information for you. Word of mouth is the best form of advertising and asking around could help you narrow down the choices better.

Wishing You All The Best

Your new exercise program doesn't have to last more than a half-hour to an hour, three or four days per week. That's a small amount of time to set aside in order to have a healthy lifestyle. A *little* is better than nothing and you will *always* feel better afterwards even if it's just the peace of mind for doing something. Think about how many hours you spend on the couch watching TV or on other meaningless tasks that you won't benefit from.

Just be patient and let yourself adapt to the changes you are making. My best recommendation is to always finish your workout with the feeling that you can do more. This will keep you from wearing yourself out too much and 'burning out' before you give yourself a real chance to begin. Don't let your enthusiasm get the best of you either. I admit being guilty of getting too excited about something and over-doing it.

I hope I was able to answer some important questions for you in order to help you get started. I wish you all the best in your exciting adventure for a healthy lifestyle.

Live Healthy – Be Free,

Tony Simoneli

P.S. Don't forget to read the bonuses that I've included.

Resources

Centers for Disease Control & Prevention – www.cdc.gov

Department of Health and Human Services – www.hhs.gov

Journal of the American Medical Association – www.jamia.org

American Medical Association – www.ama-assn.org

National Center for Health Statistics –
www.cdc.gov/nchs/index.htm

National Academy of Sports Medicine – www.nasm.org

Personal Fitness Professional – www.fit-pro.com

Web MD – www.webmd.com

Bonuses

There is so much that I could add to the book but I felt it would have become too overwhelming if I was to include everything that I thought would be useful. However, if you would like to have some extra bonuses to help you reach your goals email me at: **StartHereBooks@gmail.com** and I'll email them to you.

LaVergne, TN USA
22 September 2010
197964LV00002B/9/P